Author and Director
Albinas Kirkilas

This book is one of the rare examples when a book is born after the movie. In September of 2015, a group of young self-taught filmmakers decided to create a project BEAT YOUR MORNING DEVIL. The idea was presented as a short film on the well-known crowd funding platform – KICKSTARTER. At first, to achieve success with this project seemed to be impossible, but when the last minutes were ticking on the crowd funding platform created a wide smile on each member of our team face. And those young smiley faces decided not to stop with a film, but also got inspired to make a book related on the film BEAT YOUR MORNING DEVIL idea. While making this film we were searching and testing the most effective tricks to "BEAT YOUR MORNING DEVIL".

In this book, you will find the best tricks to wake up on time that we have found and tested in half a year. Some of the tips focus on how to prepare to go to sleep, some of them focus on the sleeping process itself, and some help in extreme situations, when you are in desperate need to wake up, but you have not got enough sleep. We promise that not only you will find ideas how to beat your own morning devil, but you will also be inspired to find your own ways how to get rid of the beast.

1 Find a responsible friend who runs in the mornings (in most cases it's a lonely introvert). Your Morning Devil will have no chances when a worried introvert keeps buzzing the doorbell. P.S. Exercising is also a good thing (for many reasons).

2 Find a good reason to wake on time. If you NEED to go to work or university – it's not the best motive. But if you WANT to be the first to say happy birthday for your friend, or to watch a new episode of Game Of Thrones or to have morning sex... Your Morning Devil has no chances.

3 Use an app called ALARMY. You can set it so that the alarm stops only after taking a picture of your chosen place, for example a bathroom. P.S. Don't use this trick for longer than a week or two. Your Morning Devil might get so pissed that he will throw your precious smart phone straight to the wall.

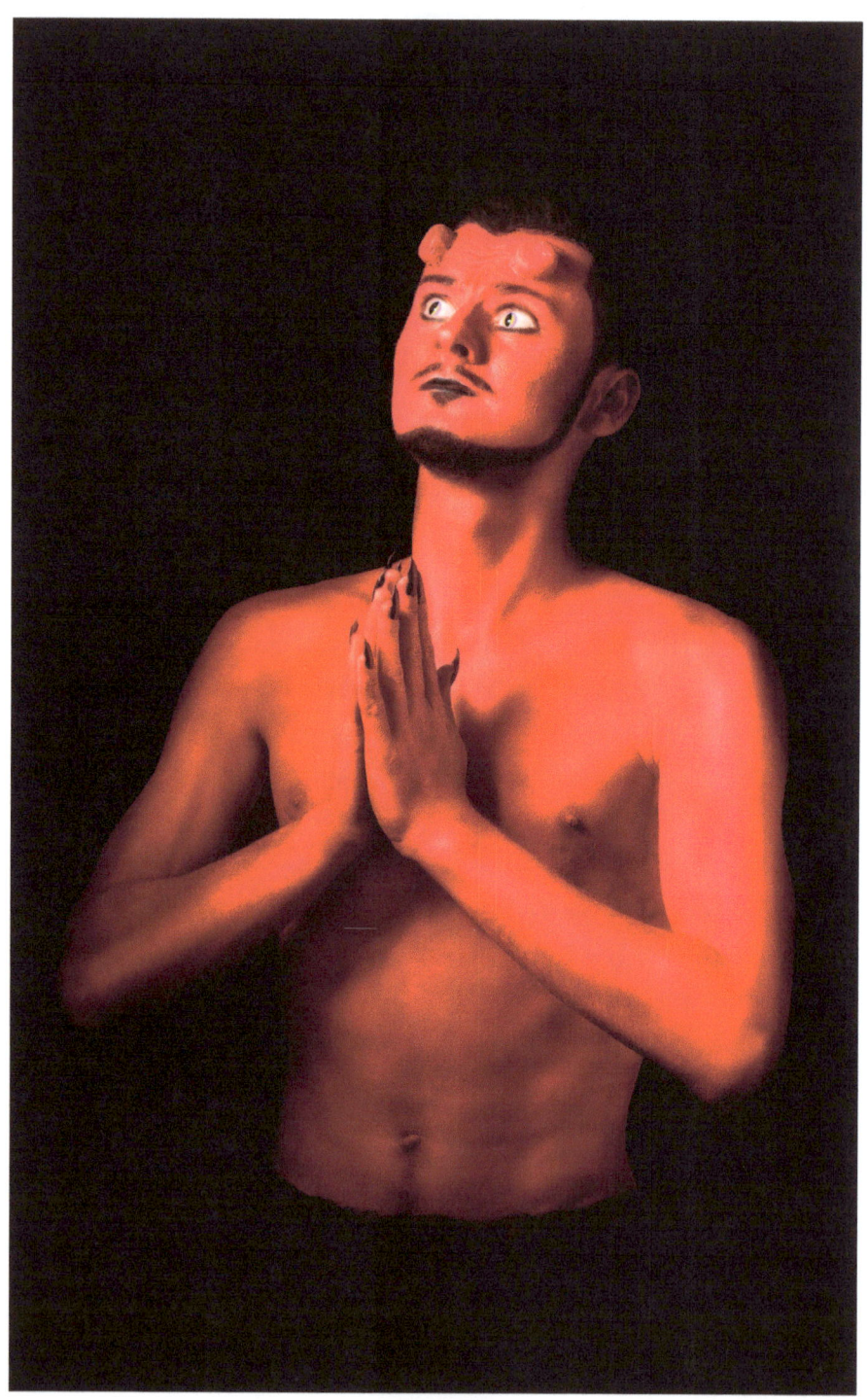

4

Have you ever heard of success chain? Here is how it works: every morning when you wake up on time, you mark an X on the calendar. A line of X'es creates a chain which itself motivates to continue the good work. Statistically, in 5 or 6 days your Morning Devil will make you break the chain, but 5 successful mornings is also a trophy. Maybe you can do more?

Ever heard of success chain?

Try an extreme routine!

5

Try an extreme routine. If your wake up time is 06: 00 and you need an hour to prepare, set your alarm on 05: 25. You can guess what will happen. Let's see if your Morning Devil can deal with it.

Have you ever heard of sleep cycles? Your Morning Devil definitely has (in his worst nightmares). The idea is that during sleep we go through a 90-minutes-long sleep cycle, which consists of transition to sleep, light sleep, deep sleep and REM sleep. To skip all the „smart stuff" about sleeping stages, all you need to know is that if you wake up on light sleep stage, it will be much easier to beat your Morning Devil than waking after 30 extra minutes of sleep. The fun part is that you don't need to count in which stage of sleep you are. You can just download one of sleep cycle apps, for example "SLEEP CYCLE". Your Morning Devil will cry like a little girl.

Ever heard of sleep cycles?

7

Do you like Coffee?

Do you like coffee? Your Morning Devil hates it. Scientists have tested a theory on rats and have found that a sniff of coffee activates several parts in the brain that in turn reduces the effort of sleep deprivation. You can test the theory by getting a coffee machine with a timer: place it within sniffing distance and set it to start brewing 10 minutes before your alarm goes off.

8

Give your friend 100€

Give your friend 100 Euros. You have read it right. Don't worry. You will get them back (probably). Every day you wake up on time your friend (or a relative) should give you 10 Euros back. If you wake up on time for 10 days, you'll get your money back. Motivation grows tremendously when it costs to be late!

9

This one works only if you don't have a big sleep debt. To tell you the truth, you have alarm not only on your bedroom drawer, but you also have one inside your body (it's called a biological clock and your Morning Devil knows nothing about it). The game is simple: before going to sleep, imagine on what time you want to wake up. Imagine how you open your eyes, look into your ceiling, and smile. Imagine how you get up for a wonderful day. The key is to trust yourself that you will wake on time without an alarm clock. Trust means you don't prepare a plan B, you are just 120% sure that you will wake up on time. Simple as that.

*Be 120%
sure that you
will wake up
on time*

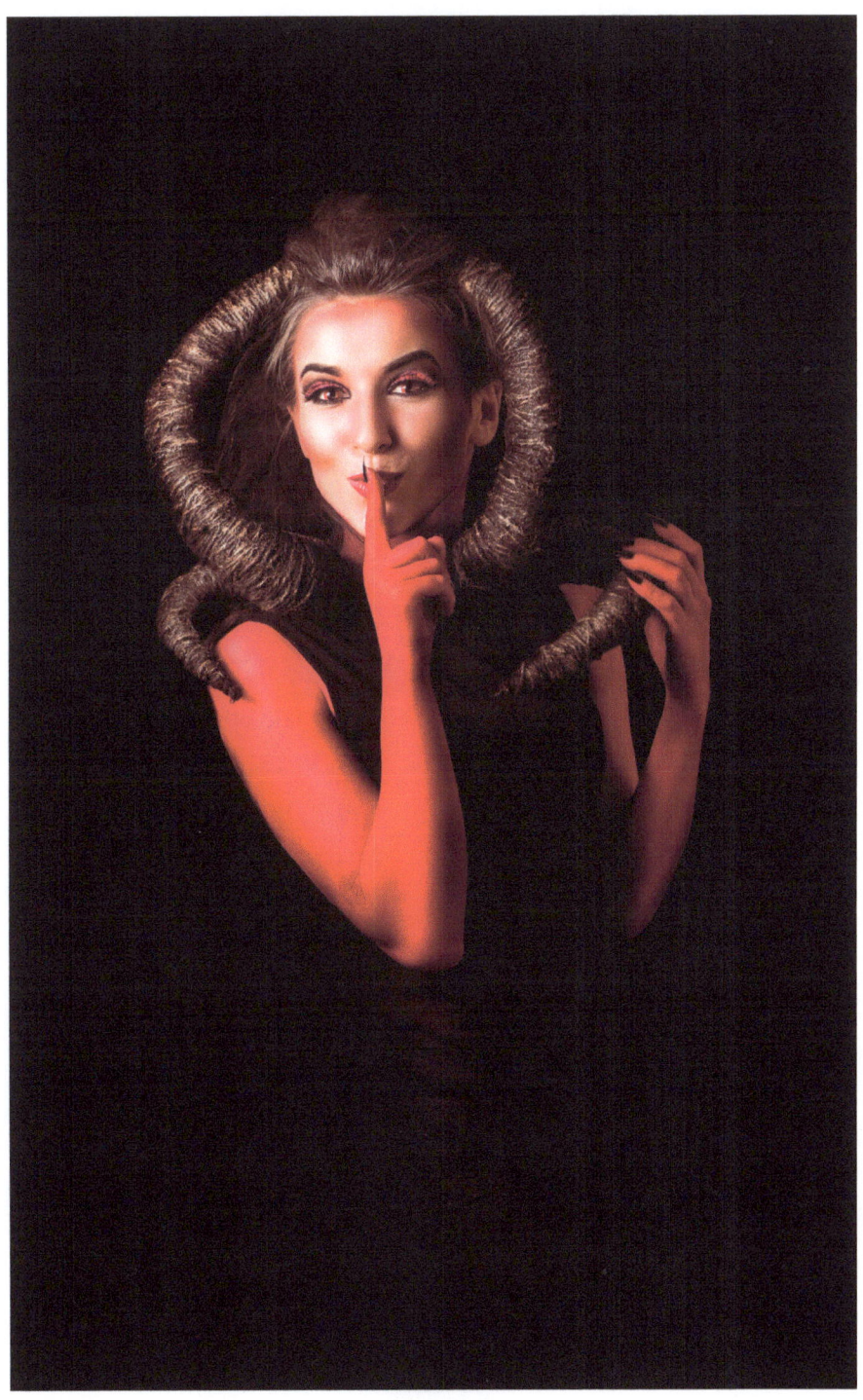

Play some loud music

One of the Morning Devil's biggest fears is loud music. If you want to beat your Morning Devil in a second or two, make your salon speakers play a song that makes you orgasm on a dance floor. A tip for volume – if you can wake you neighbors, this means the volume is just right. If you love classic films, check out film "Groundhog Day" (1993) and steal its idea of the best morning song (" I got you babe").

10

11

From a first sight, your Morning Devil may seem to be a very cruel creature. But on the other hand, he has some sensitive weaknesses. For example, sensitivity to light. Try going to sleep without closing your curtains (first make sure your neighbors do not see what they shouldn't see). This works only if the Sun hits your room on time you need to wake up. If not, try asking your relatives to turn your room lights when they hear how your Morning Devil hits the snooze button. Risky, but worth trying.

Sleep without closing curtains

Put your alarm far from your bed

If we look at your Morning Devil from the biological side, his hands are as long as your hands. This means that if your alarm clock is close enough to your bed, your Morning Devil will reach it and press the cursed snooze button. So make it a longer distance. If your alarm clock is on the other side of your room, your Morning Devil will probably be too lazy to get up and you will have another motive to get out of the bed.

12

13

Never use the same alarm clock sound for longer than three days! Your Morning Devil will get used to it. Try to wary between genres, rhythms, and speed of the alarm sounds. Remember, that it mustn't be music all the time. It can be some strange noise, maybe a soundtrack from the Comedy Club or your favorite porn film?

Use different alarm sounds

The most common Morning Devil's strategy to make you stay in bed for eternity is making your room to feel like it's in Antarctica. You move your blanket a little bit and it's so freezing that you tend to get back to the sweet dream. But there's a solution. You should be a lazy sportsman. Start from your eyes: do some exercise for your eyes. Firstly, blink as quickly as you can for 30 seconds. Then draw circles on your ceiling with your eyes (at least 20 circles in different directions). Then start spinning your wrists and other parts of your body. In 5 minutes think of getting up again.

14

15

Morning Devils can't do what they promise to do. But you can. Promise at least 5 important people that you will beat your Morning Devil for 3 or 5 days. Maybe some of them can even give you a prize if you succeed?

Make
promise to
important
people

Whether you have had a party before sleep, or not, you should consider having a glass of water next to your alarm clock. Not only does drinking water get you doing something physical (taking a glass from the drawer or walking to the kitchen), it also supplies the body with its most precious resource after a 6-8 hour drought. Drinking cooler water also helps wake up the body because of the additional energy required to heat the water during digestion. Keep in mind, it will not beat your tricky Morning Devil, but it can make the fight to be easier.

16

Consider having a glass of water

17

Your Morning Devil can name at least 15 reasons why he wants you to stay in bed after the wake up alarm rings. Can you name at least 15 reasons why you want to wake up on time? It looks like a worthless game, but you will be surprised how effective it is. Just take a blank sheet of paper and a pen. Before going to sleep write down 20 – 30 reasons why it's important to wake up on time for you. If you can't, maybe you are wasting your time trying to wake up early?

18

This one is for a bad ass. If your Morning Devil has immunity for all kinds of shocking tricks, try beating him with pleasure. Morning masturbation. This is it. You will probably lose some time, but it will definitely increase your blood flow and a little quickie will get you on your feet quicker than the snoozing era.

19

Do you have any pets? We hope you do. Especially the ones, that can touch your Morning Devil with a giant tongue or hit his feet with sharp claws. Just ask your relatives or roommates to let those little friends into your room on your wake up time.

Do you have any pets?

20

Prepare yourself a dream breakfast

Some people eat to live while some live to eat. If you fall under the food lovers' category, you should consider preparing yourself a dream breakfast. Maybe a fruit-filled tortilla or caramel pancakes? You will probably overeat, but fighting your Morning Devil demands some loses, doesn't it?

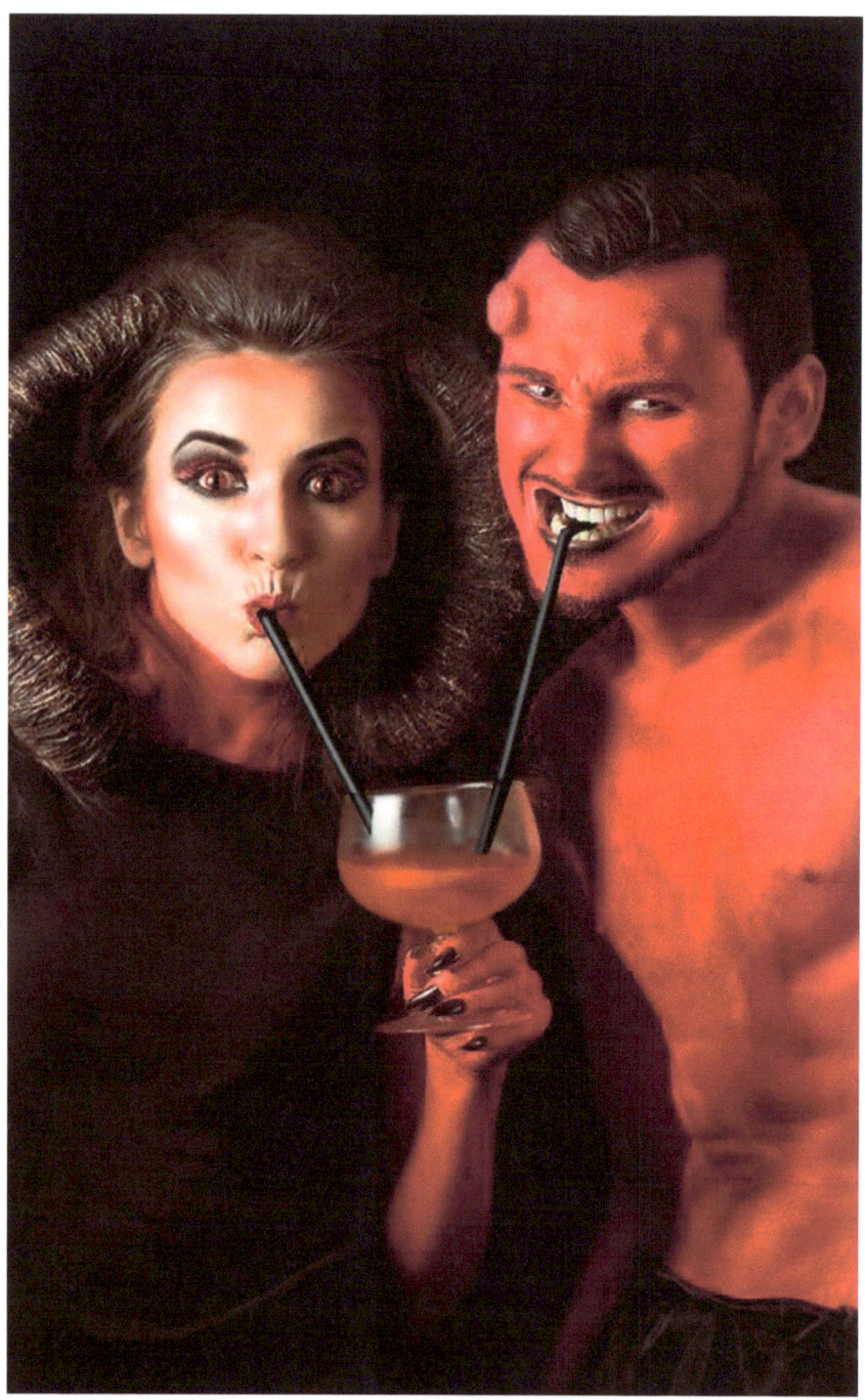

21

The 21st tip has some magic itself. You have probably heard that if you do something for 21 days, it will become a habit. We could argue whether it becomes a habit or not, but if you manage to beat your Morning Devil for 21 days, it will definitely become easier than ever before. In order to not to let your Morning Devil get into your comfort zone, try using different wake up tricks for 21 days. The main thing to remember is to keep up with the same routine even on the weekends, because exceptions will bring you back to the starting point. To add some motivation, remember Chinese proverb: "No one who can rise before dawn for 360 days a year fails to make his family rich."

Some magic of number 21

22

Check all new morning activities in your hometown. Maybe there's something worth defeating the Morning Devil? For example, a group of tai chi lovers who start their thing on sunrise.

23

Here are so many tricks to beat your Morning Devil, but maybe you don't need any of them? Maybe your will power is strong enough to get out of bed after the alarm rings? The will power also has its limits, but it's worth trying.

The biggest fear of all kinds of Morning Devils is cold shower. Unfortunately, it's probably also the biggest fear for you too. If you manage to get out of bed for a morning pee, try splashing some cold water on your face. While fighting against the Morning Devils, it's good to have at least one part of the body already wide awake.

24

Ask a person to give you a lift. This is a sneaky little trick (but sneaky tricks are the best when fighting your Morning Devil). If you share lifts to work, then you'll be forced to get up on time in the morning. You won't want to let your fellow commuter down, or make them late. You'll also pick up a bit more on the way to work; you'll behave chirpier because it's rude to be distant and ignorant around other people.

25

26

Keep a wake up experience log and evaluate it weekly. Keep track of all the tricks you use and give an honest feedback of what is working for you and what is not. Do you have more energy? A peppier mood? Are you more patient with your family? Or maybe your Morning Devil still wins the fight? After you've tried a new strategy or two for a week, take a look at your journal. If the steps you're taking are working, keep it up. If not, take another look at the obstacles and think, maybe there can be some changes that your Morning Devil will not tolerate. Be self-compassionate as you learn how to make this important lifestyle change.

27

Become a lazy yoga professional! An Oxford University study found that pranayama or yoga breathing "had a markedly invigorating effect on perceptions of both mental and physical energy and increased high positive mood." The most common form is called Three Part Breath or Dirgha Breath. You can do it lying in bed: Inhale deeply through your nose, filling up belly. Expand your belly like a balloon. Continue to inhale, expanding ribs like gills on a fish. When you are completely full, empty yourself slowly but completely, exhaling through your nose. Do six to ten rounds. If it sounds difficult, watch a Youtube tutorial. Your Morning Devil will be blown away!

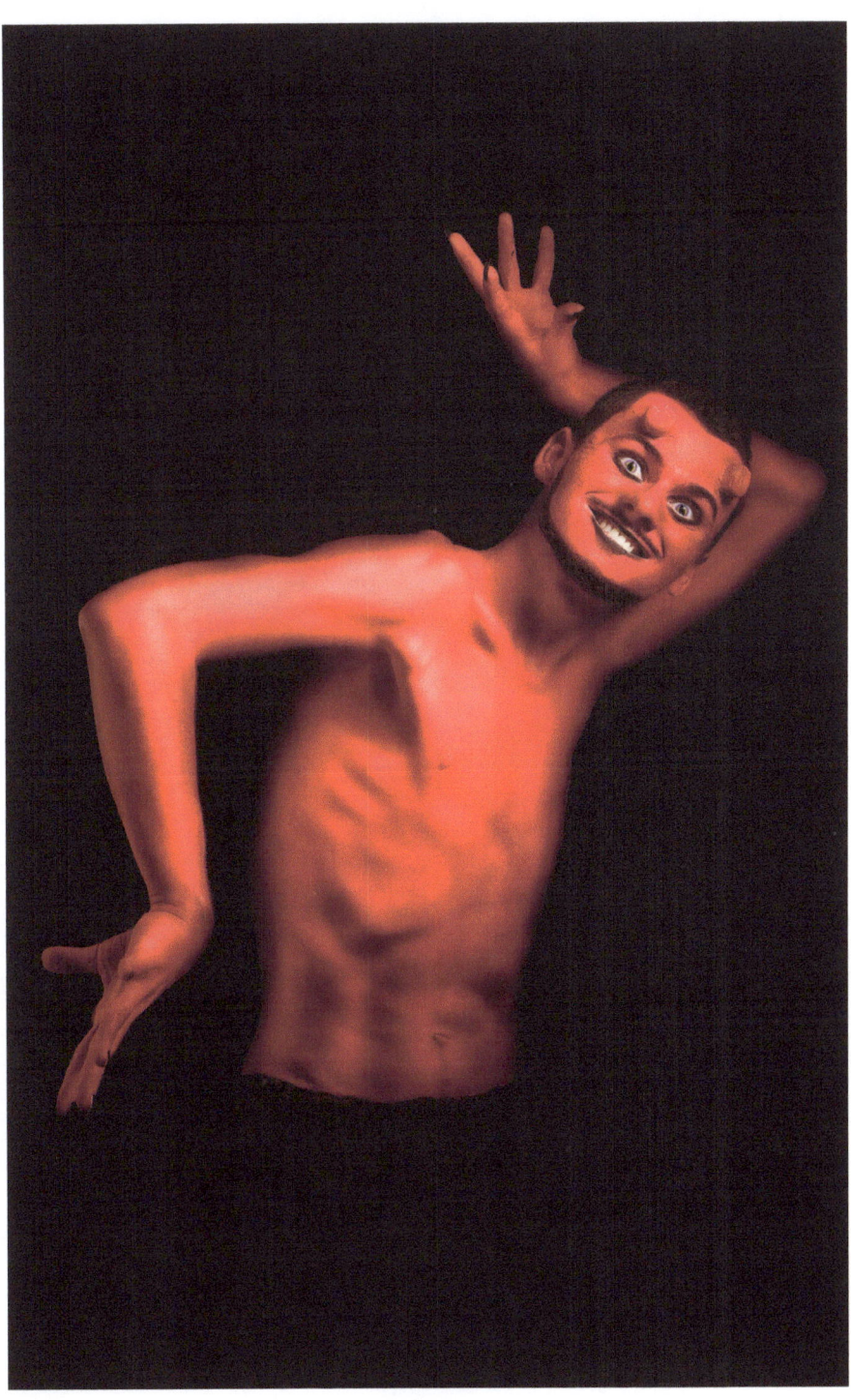

Not only Morning Devil tries to make your sleep destroy your day. Food, drink, medication, stress, television, and digital devices are just a few of the things that can contribute to tossing and turning. What else keeps you up? The temperature? Light? Noise? Work to create an optimal sleeping environment by eliminating the things that are getting in the way.

28

Do you like eating frogs? You should! Many famous success psychology lectors name your most important tasks of the day as a frog. Usually, at first sight it seems to be as unpleasant experience as eating a frog. Usually those tasks are very hard to do, very responsible and time consuming. But it's very healthy to make them to be the first thing to do on your day. It's easy for your Morning Devil to make you oversleep some unimportant meeting, but it's much harder when you go to sleep in the mood to start the morning from something very important. In most cases, it isn't fun, but usually, if you manage to do the task successfully, the other part of the day will be fun as hell.

29

30

This one is a little bit risky, but worth trying. Try sleeping in another place. Some theory says it's even better to sleep on the ground. There are a few advantages: by doing this you are leaving your comfort zone, maybe even your Morning Devil. The risk is that it may be much harder to fall asleep in a different place.

31

Homework that might save your day (must be done before sleep). Take a piece of paper and write all the things that you need to do in your life. It doesn't matter how big or small they are. They might vary from washing your socks to graduating from college. Thinking on starting French classes? Write that down. Going to a birthday party on Saturday? Write that down and write that you will go to buy a present. Everything that you can think of, everything you was about to forget. Check every blinking light in your head and make a sentence out of it. Usually grown-ups write from 100 to 200 things they need to do. The trick is that after doing it you will feel less stress (there's nothing to forget). Another advantage – your inner motivation environment changes at 100 percent. And that's the worst nightmare of your sleepy friend.

32

One good thing to know – your body produces melatonin only when it's dark in the room. But is it really dark when you sleep? Maybe your TV's, computer mouse or some other lights are blinking? You can either turn those things off or cover their lights. Better sleep makes the fight easier to win.

33

If you wake up unprepared and there's a lazy Morning Devil laying on your back, you have one last chance. Think of the most positive thing you'll be doing that day. Is it worth to risk oversleeping?

34

Who said that it's hot in hell? Morning Devils are used to lower your room temperature in the morning to make it more difficult for you to wake up. If this is possible, , set your thermostat so that your room becomes a few degrees warmer 30 minutes prior to your alarm going off. When we wake up, our core temperature rises, while when our core body temperature lowers (you know the reason), we are sleepy. When you wake up in the morning, the ideal room temperature for your body should be 22 degrees.

Improve waking time with patience

Fight against your Morning Devil may become much easier if you have time and patience. If you always wake up at 10 ~ 11 am, it may be not realistic to expect that you will immediately beat your Morning Devil at 5 am the next day (unless you have bigger balls than your Morning Devil). Start off by improving your waking time by 15 ~ 30 mins every day until you reach your goal.

35

36

Have you ever thought what will you get if you beat your Morning Devil? If you wake up for some compelling reason – it's fine. If not – think again. Scientists have proved that the best motivation is not when you are about to get punished, neither when you get a prize. Best motivation is when it's a combination of both. So what reward will you give yourself if you manage to beat your Morning Devil?

Wake up for some compelling reason

Make your goals visible

37

Embed your goal consciously and subconsciously into your mind. If you have a notice board, you can put up your goals on the board. Any kind of visual that reminds you how important it is to beat your Morning Devil for you. Other options are to stick it up on a post-it note in front of your computer or set it as your wallpaper.

38

Generate motivation with a friend

Work on the goal with someone else. If you have a friend who also has a goal to beat his Morning Devil this will help to generate more motivation to wake up earlier.

39

This one never works, but maybe you are some kind of magician. It's a secret technique that has been tested for ages. Rumors say that Morning Devils can't do anything against this technique, unfortunately, nobody yet succeeded to test this technique. The technique is called GOING TO SLEEP EARLIER. Maybe you are the one who can do it once and for all.

40

Get out of the bed immediately once you hear the alarm. We all know how it feels in the morning when we wake up. The Devil's voice in our head is just coaxing to go back to sleep every morning despite our best intents to wake up. Instead of giving it the chance to speak, haul yourself out of your bed the second the alarm rings. While you may feel like the lead for the first 5 ~ 10 minutes, the Morning Devil will start wearing off beyond that. Before you know it, you will be awake and ready to start the day.

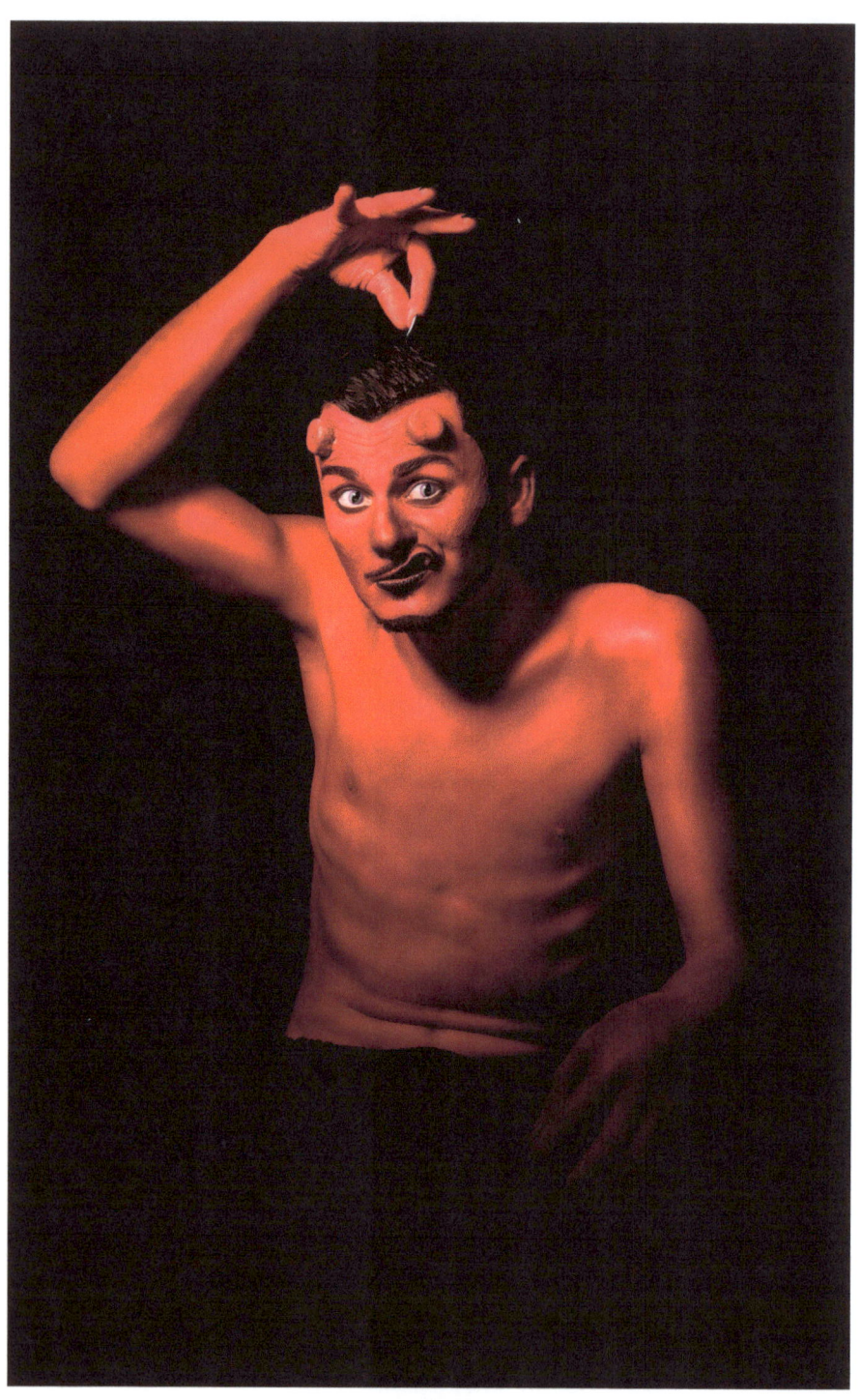

*Make
an early
date*

*Get a
white noise
machine*

*Make
your bed
comfortable*

41

Consider getting a white noise machine. Many people find the sounds from white noise machines to be very soothing. Our brains are wired to wake up when we heard random noises. Having a white noise machine "gives the brain a tonic signal that dampens its own internal systems," says Dr. Ralph Pascualy, the medical director of Northwest Hospital Sleep Center in Seattle.

42

Take an early date. You wouldn't be late for that, would you? And meeting at sunrise together may be even more romantic than anything you are used to do in the evening... Even if you don't have a partner yet, or if the magic person also has problems with their Morning Devil, maybe you can do some kind of romantic surprise? Like gluing his or her car with lots of smiley faces before he leaves to collage/ work.

43

Maybe bad mattress is one of the reasons why your Morning Devil still manages to win? Make your bed comfortable. If you need to get a new mattress, consider buying or saving up for one. Remember that you spend 1/ 3 of your life in bed, and the quality of your sleep impacts the other 2/ 3 in a major way.

44

Sleeping can be some kind of experience itself. Check up your local crazy people. Maybe there's someone who organizes a gong night, where a bunch of people got to sleep in their sleeping bags while a few gong gurus keep playing the gong for the whole night. Or maybe a group of old hippies organize lucid dreaming night, when you go to sleep while listening to a sound that should help you to have a lucid dream? Your Morning Devil will definitely never visit places like this, but for you it's a treasure – new experience, new environment, and a guarantee that you will not oversleep.

*Cool stuff
for waking up
on Ebay*

45

If you have both, the Morning Devil and showing off the Devil, you should check out the cool stuff for waking up early that you can find on Ebay. One of examples is a flying alarm clock. The idea is that it takes of playing some loud sound and will definitely not stop till you catch it.

The National Sleep Foundation has some statistics that may change your sleeping duration forever. Check how much you actually need to sleep to live a healthy and happy life.

46

Newborns (0-3 months):	Infants (4-11 months):	Toddlers (1-2 years):
Sleep range narrowed to 14-17 hours each day (previously it was 12-18)	Sleep range widened two hours to 12-15 hours (previously it was 14-15)	Sleep range widened by one hour to 11-14 hours (previously it was 12-14)
Preschoolers (3-5):	**School age children (6-13):**	**Teenagers (14-17):**
Sleep range widened by one hour to 10-13 hours (previously it was 11-13)	Sleep range widened by one hour to 9-11 hours (previously it was 10-11)	Sleep range widened by one hour to 8-10 hours (previously it was 8.5-9.5)
Younger adults (18-25):	**Adults (26-64):**	**Older adults (65+)**
Sleep range is 7-9 hours (new age category)	Sleep range did not change and remains 7-9 hours	Sleep range is 7-8 hours (new age category)

47

Take a bath to rise your body's temperature a few degrees before going to sleep. The cooling down phase after the bath mimics your body's natural temperature drop in the evening, relaxing you. Better sleep – easy fight.

48

You may need to take a look at your diet. Having a light dinner (or even fasting for around 16 hours before wake-up time) can help you readjust your wake up routine. Avoid caffeine or other stimulants, which can take 5 to 10 hours to work their way through your body, in the evening. Likewise, avoid depressants, such as alcohol, because they slow down your metabolism, which messes up your sleep cycle. What types of things help you get better sleep? Making sure you get some exercise over the course of your day can help you sleep better at night! Doing 20 to 40 minutes of aerobic exercise at least four days a week can improve your sleep quality.

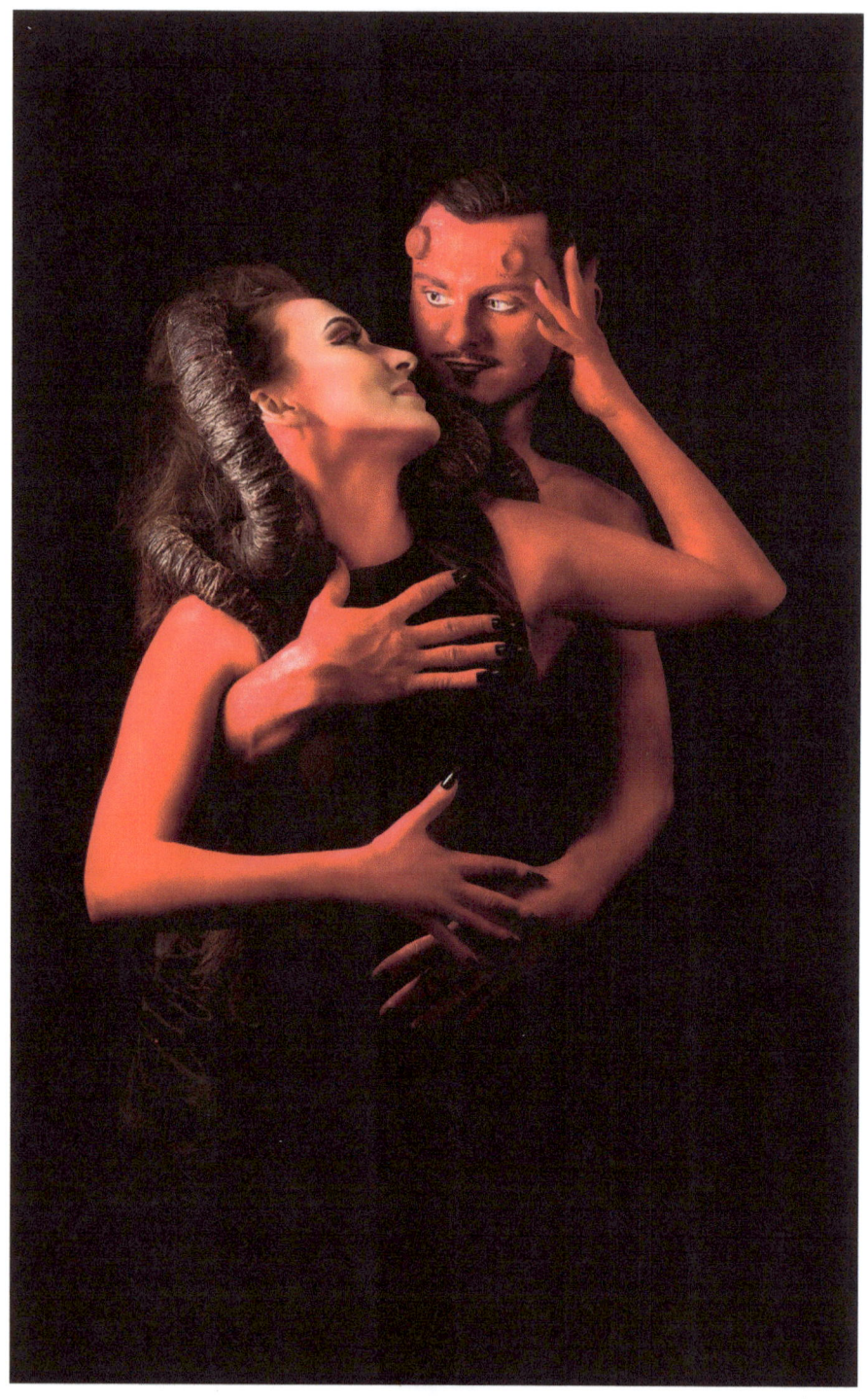

49

One of the biggest dilemmas in life is whether it's worth going to sleep when you have to wake up in 40 minutes or not. In most cases sleep experts suggest to go to sleep, but if you have a chance you may try both solutions. As a matter of fact, if you don't go to sleep, you do not risk to be beaten by your Morning Devil (still, keep in mind that your health is priority number 1).

50

According to the National Sleep Foundation, light and the absence of light are essential indicators to our brains of when we should be asleep and when we should be awake. Simply put, darkness means it's time to sleep, and light means it's time to wake up. Studies have shown that the light emitted from electronic devices, including televisions, tablets, and cell phones, is enough to disrupt our natural rhythms of sleep and wakefulness. So put away your electronics for an hour before you go to bed, and wind down with a book instead. Beat your Morning Devil before the morning fight.

51

Call your mom. It sounds strange, but a conversation with your mother is bound to wake you up. Possibly, it's the deep emotional connection to the woman who woke you up for years. Regardless of your current relationship, either the stress or the charm of calling her will get you going. Besides, she probably thinks you don't call her enough anyway, so it couldn't hurt.

52

Not only does the early bird get the worm, he's generally happier and has a higher overall satisfaction with his life. "We don't know why this is, but there are a few potential explanations. Evening people may be more prone to social jet lag; this means that their biological clock is out of sync with the social clock," Renee Biss, a researcher wrote in a study conducted by the University of Toronto. You have just read some argument about why it is good to beat your Morning Devil. You should read more. Google for more information, why it is worth waking up on time. Information will help you with motivation. It's like a fear of spiders. Most people fear spiders, especially tarantulas, but usually after gathering more information about spiders they even manage to touch those cute little creatures.

53

Brush your teeth with peppermint toothpaste. The smell of peppermint stimulates your body's trigeminal nerve, giving you an energy boost. Brushing your teeth with peppermint toothpaste first thing is a great way to perk up. Do it before you have anything to eat, since brushing immediately after eating isn't very good for your teeth. This trick will not get you out of the bed quicker, but it will definitely make sure you will not go back to bed.

Peppermint toothpaste gives an energy

Sleep on the right side

54

They say that if everything isn't going right, you should go left. Not when it comes to sleeping. Another way to have a better sleep is to do it on the right side. Research has suggested that sleeping on your right side has a positive influence on dreams, decreasing mood dysfunction during the day.

55

Pull your hair. This one sounds bad but it really isn't; slowly and gently tug at your hair to get blood flowing to your head in a new and refreshing way. It's not as drastic as most of the other tricks in this book, but if you're just feeling the beginning tinges of sleepiness, it can help. Besides, it's better to pull your hair by yourself than by your Morning Devil.

Pull your hair to get blood flowing

56

Embrace the power of silence

Embrace silence. Silence is usually needed to go to sleep initially; however, sleeping while some music is playing in the background prevents our fore brain from resting and contributes to sleep deprivation. It's okay for a night or two, but not a longer perspective.

57

If you are a social networks addict and you are popular there – use it. Make your computer turn on automatically and work as an alarm clock. It should turn on your beloved social network, so that you would be convinced by news, likes, comments and shares. Also there's an app which posts something naughty on you facebook if your snooze button is touched. Bad trick for a life time, but a day or two is worth trying.

58

Pop a strong mint: The stronger the better because the effervescent effects do a great job of waking you up. If you're on the verge of narcolepsy, consider getting a menthol stick— they're so strong that they help actors fake tears. A pack of them could be laying next to your alarm clock.

59

If you have managed to leave your home but you still feel that the Morning Devil is following you, try social interaction with a complete stranger. This is one that nobody ever thinks about until after it's already happened by accident. If you're feeling dead on your feet, mention something about the weather to someone nearby. Acting tired is no big deal in front of friends, but our bodies tend to wake up pretty quickly to avoid any sort of social awkwardness.

If you are a social networks addict...

Consider getting a menthol stick

Try social interaction with a stranger

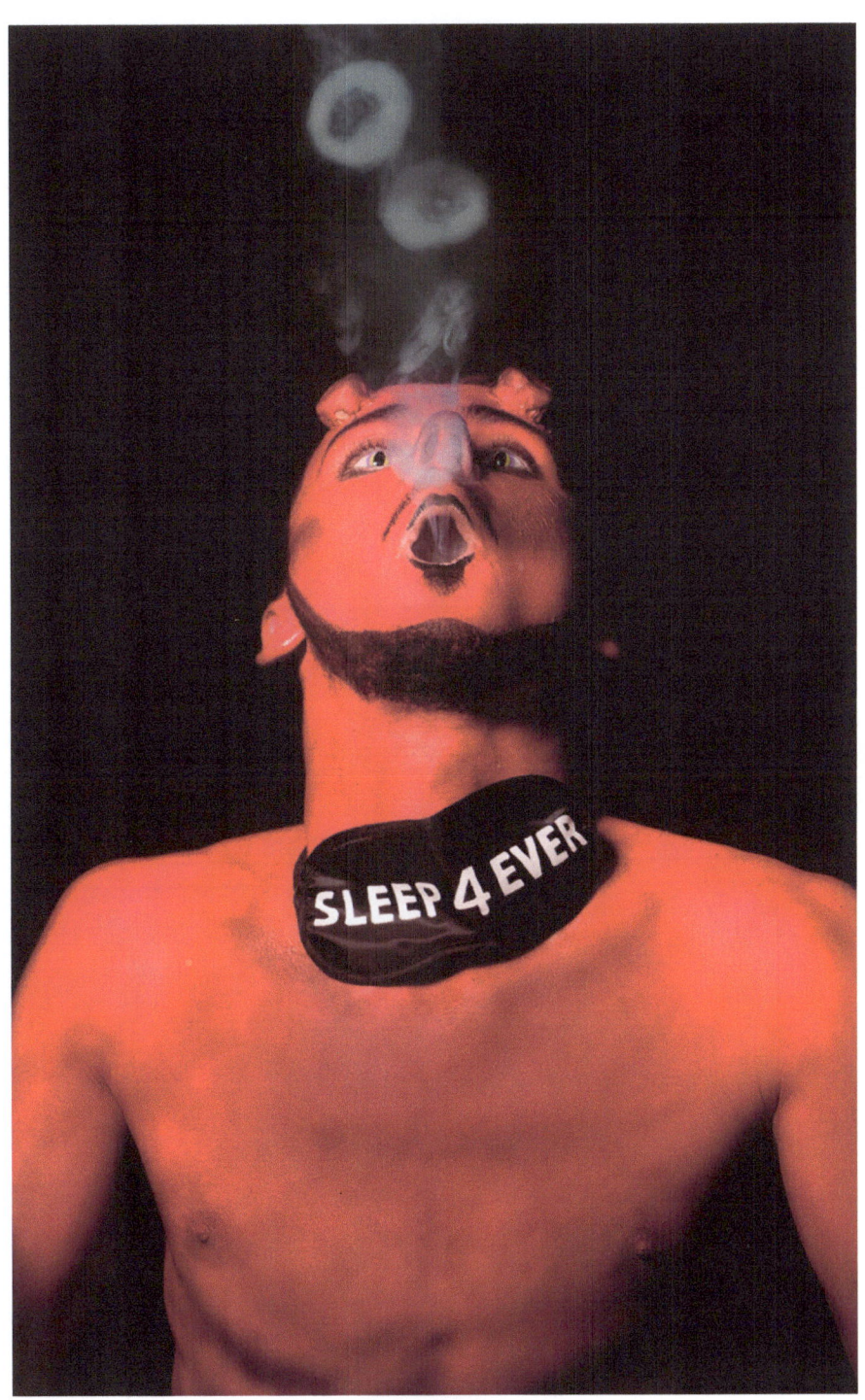

60

Bite a lemon! Whether you like the sour fruit or not, you can't deny the zesty slap to the face that it can provide in a time of need.

61

Pick your outfit the night before. This is advice that everybody knows, but it actually helps. Nothing is worse than having to wake up early and then only having fifteen minutes to choose your outfit and pull your life together. By having an outfit you're excited and ready to go, you'll want to get up and get ready. It also saves time, which allows you to get your life together a little easier.

62

Do you have lots of stuff on your ceiling? No? Then there's something you might glue there. Steal pictures from Google that illustrate you biggest goals. Want a new car? Get a picture. Want to be a basketball champion? Get a picture. Want to have a nice butt? Get a picture. Just anything you want. Glue them to your ceiling. The most important part – don't look at those pictures unless you have just heard your alarm clock.

63

If visualization wasn't crazy enough for you, then this may sound as a killer. But try at least once to make sure whether it's nonsense or some sort of magic. The idea is simple. After you hear the alarm ring, allow your Morning Devil to turn it off and start with repeating the same phrase (loudly): I AM A WONDERFUL PERSON, I WILL GET OUT OF BED NOW AND HAVE AN AMAZING DAY. Repeat for 20 times, louder and louder. No questions, just try it. And it's not only about beating your Morning Devil.

64

Sleep with fresh air. It's vital to understand that deep, relaxing sleep is one of key ways to easy wakeup. Quite often you may sleep for 10 hours straight yet feel drowsy in the morning. There may be many reasons for that, and stale or stuffy air, or even fats of your Morning Devil could be one of them. Open the windows, get more fresh air in the room and enjoy the sleeping! If you live in the place where you prefer not to open the windows, get an air refreshener and revitalizer . You'll feel the difference once wake up refreshed and then feel energetic all day. One more way to increase oxygen level in your body is taking a walk outside before going to sleep. Those of you who have dogs and walk them every evening know how it works. These tips are highly recommended to the people suffering from insomnia.

65

If lavender and chamomile soothe, why not use your olfactory system to become alert? Another out-of-the-ordinary alarm clock is the Peaceful Progression Alarm Clock, which uses timed aromatherapy emissions as well as light and noise to wake you. That may not be a quick and cheap solution for most people, but essential oils can be. Lemon, lime, grapefruit, juniper, and ginger are all known to have energizing properties, while rosemary, basil, black pepper, and peppermint help mental clarity. Fight your morning drag with a timed diffuser, personal aromatherapy inhaler, roll-on aromatherapy device, candle, or even a scented tissue to sniff. Just be careful when mixing your own essential oils; they're powerfully concentrated and can be dangerous to your skin and children.

66

Shake it till you make it. Another amazing alarm app turns off only when you shake it hard enough! The good news is that while shaking your phone your Morning Devil will fall of your back. Just type in app each „shake alarm" and choose the right one for you.

66,6

Become friends with your Morning Devil. Fighting from the beggining of your day can be really entertaining, but even more entertaining can be waking up in peace and happiness. Of course, to achieve this trick is much harder than any other trick in this book. But if you spent some time to find how to find what you have in common with your devil, results may be marvelous. If you both have the same goal in the morning, and it's not sleeping, then your will definatelly live a Chinese proverb say in this book.

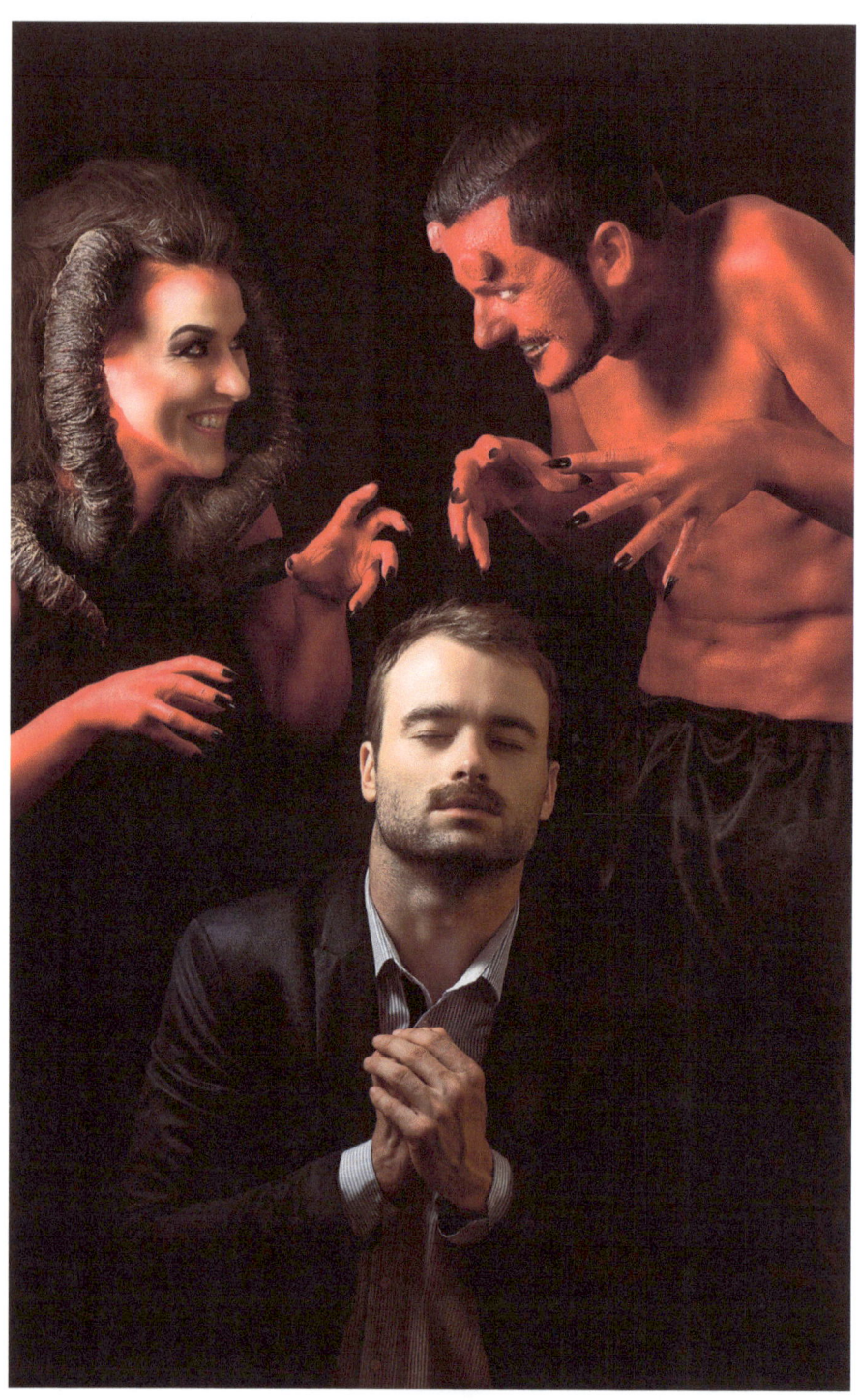

Now you are ready.

You are ready to meet your Morning Devil again and show him a surprise or two. We wish you to succeed on waking up on time because it's an amazing experience when after the first part of the the day you have already achieved a few personal victories. You are already proud of yourself and you are prepared for new projects. To tell you a secret, we are also ready for new projects. We want to meet our inner devil again. The idea is still hidden under 10 locks from any attention, but we can say that it will not be about waking up on time any more. We have much more inner fights that we sometimes don't even notice. We will take another look at them from a different perspective. As people say, when you notice your problem, you have half of victory already. So if you are interested in another game with the inner guy or gal that usually has a different opinion than you, follow our process on facebook: BEAT YOUR MORNING DEVIL. It would be great if you could share examples of your personal fight with a Morning Devil. Thank you for your support and see you in a very close future.